CW00665987

PILATES BAR

EXERCISE

Unlock Your Body's Potential and Achieve Total Body Transformation with the Power of Pilates Bar Workouts for Beginners

By

AMANDA GILBERT

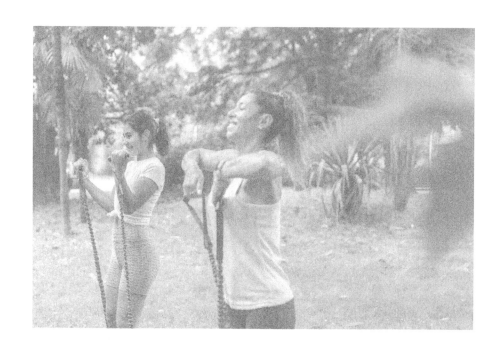

CONTENTS

Introduction

INTRODUCTION

Your strength and flexibility can be improved using the Pilates bar exercises. These workouts can be done at home with basic equipment, making them the perfect option for those who want to get in shape but don't have access to a gym. Pilate's bars are great for improving posture and strengthening your core muscles. They can also be used to strengthen your arms, legs, and back. If you are new to Pilates, it is advisable to take a few classes with a trained teacher before performing any of the exercises at home. Once you fully understand the foundations, you may experiment with different exercises and exercise combinations to find the ones that work best for you. Always remember that there is no one-size-fits-all approach to fitness, so pick an exercise routine you enjoy and that is tailored to your individual requirements.

A Pilates bar will help you advance your training if you choose to practice Pilates in the convenience of your own home.

The Pilates bar is one of the instruments that might improve your workout, even if Pilates doesn't require any special equipment. In essence, the bar gives your movements more resistance, which heightens their effectiveness.

The idea is similar to resistance bands if you've ever used them. During your Pilates practice, the bar uses elasticized bands that combine with your body weight to intensify your movements.

Do Pilates Bars Work

If you choose the appropriate set, Pilates bars can be a simple (and reasonably priced) way to maximize your mat time and ensure that you feel the burn.

Investing in one of these bars can give you an added challenge by making your workout harder than it would be only using body weight if you've been practicing Pilates for a while and feel like you've recently reached a plateau.

The bars are great for folks with limited room and those who wish to carry some exercise gear on vacation because they are portable and light enough to store easily.

The Pilates Bar Can You Build Muscle

Working out with a Pilates bar can be a terrific way to gain muscle, whether your goal is to get toned or bulk up. Pilates bars are perfect for a variety of activities because they are lightweight and simple to use. These exercises are simple to do out at home with this particular equipment.

Additionally, because they have low impact, they are kind to your joints and allow you to exercise longer and harder without placing too much strain on your body.

Additionally, the repetitious nature of Pilates exercises might eventually enhance muscle endurance.

Although the bar won't do the job for you, it can be a helpful tool for strengthening and toning particular muscle areas as well as your entire body. For instance, exercises like triceps, dips, and bicep curls can assist define your upper body while chest presses and rows can help shape and sculpt your arms.

Additionally, you may customize your workout to concentrate

specifically on the regions you wish to target thanks to the versatility of the Pilates bar. Therefore, a Pilates bar can be exactly what you need if you're seeking for a quick and effective workout. To increase muscular gains, you can also incorporate whey protein powder into your exercise regimen.

The Best Advantages of Pilates Workouts with Bars

Using the Pilates bar to exercise can help you become more flexible.

The Pilates bar is a great tool for stretching. Using a pilates bar allows you to improve your range of motion and concentrate on specific muscles. These exercises can be used by anyone who want to become more flexible but may not have the time or drive to go to a traditional gym.

There are many exercises that can be done with a pilates bar, and each one can help to increase flexibility in a different way. The standing leg lift is the best exercise for hamstring development. The exercise involves elevating one leg behind you while holding onto the bar.

A great exercise for increasing flexibility is the back extension. During this workout, the erector spine muscles, which run along the spine, are engaged. This exercise requires you to arch your back while holding onto the bar.

Flexibility and overall fitness can both be improved with Pilates bar movements. You may maximize the effectiveness of your workout and achieve notable results by focusing on a few key muscles.

You burn calories while performing Pilates bar workouts.

You may increase your flexibility and tone your muscles by doing Pilates bar workouts. The workouts are ideal for people who want to avoid using equipment because they use your body weight as resistance.

You can modify your workout to suit your demands by choosing from a range of various pilates bar workouts. Focus on exercises that target particular muscle groups if you want to tone your muscles. For instance, tricep dips work your upper arms while standing side bends aid tonify your obliques.

Concentrate on stretching your muscles if you want to increase your flexibility. For instance, the chest opener stretches your chest and shoulders while the standing hamstring stretch aids in lengthening your hamstrings. Exercises with the Pilates bar are a terrific method to increase your general health and fitness.

Pilates bar movements, coordination and strength can be improved.

Pilates bars are a fantastic exercise to increase strength and coordination. You may tone your muscles and raise your general level of fitness by applying your own body weight as resistance. Squats, lunges, crunches, and other exercises can all be performed using pilates bars.

Utilizing a Pilates bar has many advantages, including enhanced balance, coordination, and strength. Consider incorporating Pilates bars into your exercise regimen if you're seeking for a way to increase your general level of fitness. Your balance, strength, and coordination will improve immediately.

Pilates bar workouts help to improve balance.

Balance exercises using the Pilates bar are quite effective. You can concentrate on your balance and stability while executing the workout by using the bar to support your body. Those who struggle with balance will particularly benefit from this. By strengthening your core muscles, Pilates bar movements can help you balance out. While you exercise, the bar also aids in maintaining your body's alignment. This can lessen the risk of accidents and enhance your posture in general.

THE FINEST PILATES BAR EXERCISES FOR HOME USE

The top Pilates bar exercises for today are shown below. People of all fitness levels can benefit from doing Pilates bar workouts. Pilates bar exercises are a terrific choice if you're searching for a workout that can enhance your posture, tone your muscles, and aid in calorie burning.

Walking Stretch

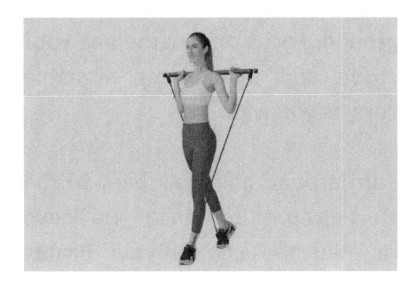

Pilates bars are an excellent way to mix up your Pilates exercises. With a Pilates bar, you can perform the straightforward but powerful exercise known as the walking stretch. Hold the Pilates bar in front of you with both hands as you stand with your feet shoulder-width apart. Move forward slowly while maintaining a straight back and the Pilates bar parallel to the ground. Focus on lengthening your stride and maintaining a stable core as you walk.

Turn around and walk back to the starting position once you have reached the end of your Pilates bar. 10-15 times should be used in this exercise. A great way to lengthen your muscles and enhance your posture is to do a walking stretch. Pilates bars are adaptable exercise tools that can be used in many different exercises. Consider using a Pilates bar if you're looking for a way to mix up your Pilates routine.

Leg Stretching

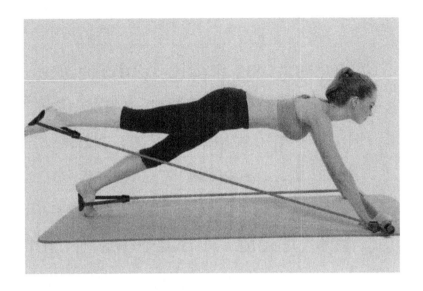

Numerous leg-stretching exercises can be done to increase the flexibility and range of motion in the legs, including Pilates Bar Leg Stretching. These exercises are convenient and inexpensive because they can be performed at home with little to no equipment.

The following are some of the best leg stretches:

1. Stretches for the hamstrings - The hamstrings are a group of large muscles in the back of the leg. Standing, sitting, and using resistance bands are all acceptable positions for hamstring stretches.
2. Stretches for the quadriceps - The quadriceps are a group of big muscles in the front of the leg.
3. Stretches for the calf - The calf is a big muscle located in the back of the lower thigh. Standing, sitting, and using

resistance bands are all acceptable ways to execute calf stretches.

4. The piriformis muscle in the buttocks, which can tighten up and create low back pain, is the focus of these exercises

5. Stretching the piriformis can be done while seated or standing, and with or without resistance bands.

These are only a handful of the numerous leg stretching exercises that may be performed to increase the legs' flexibility and range of motion. Find out which exercises are most effective for you by speaking with a physical therapist or Pilates instructor.

Barbell Exercise

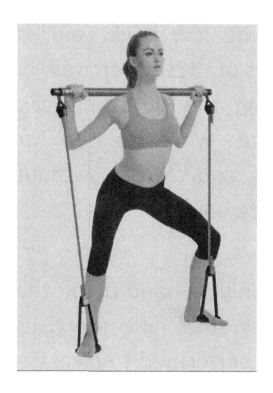

Your entire body will benefit greatly from Pilates Barbell

Exercise. For this exercise, the Pilates Bar is an excellent equipment to utilize because it offers resistance and aids in maintaining proper form. Your quads, hamstrings, glutes, core, and arms are all worked up by this workout. Start by standing with the Pilates Bar in front of you and your feet hip-width apart. Squat down by bending your knees and bringing your hips down. Be sure to maintain a straight back and a tight core. Put your heels down and stand tall from this stance. The Pilates Bar should then be raised overhead and pressed straight up into the air toward the ceiling. Make sure to maintain a tight core and a straight back during the entire movement. Pilates Barbell Exercise is a fantastic technique to work out and work out your whole body.

Waist Twisting

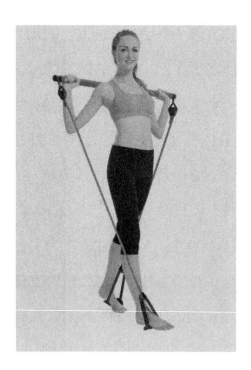

Pilates Bar Waist Twisting is a Pilates motion that serves to tone and build the abdominal muscles while also offering a gentle twisting action that can aid to decompress the spine. This motion can be performed with or without a Pilates reformer, however employing a Pilates reformer will give additional resistance and support. To perform Pilates Bar Waist Twisting, start by sitting on the Pilates reformer with your legs extended in front of you and your feet put flat against the football. Place your hands on the Pilates bar and exhale as you rotate your torso to the right, keeping your shoulders down and your core drawn in. Inhale and Ensure to repeat from the position started to your the opposite side. Include the Pilates Bar Waist Twisting in your Pilates reformer routine right away for a great ab workout and spine decompression.

Bar Kick

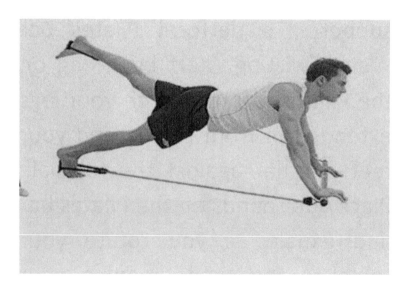

The Pilates Bar Kicks method is an excellent way to tone your legs and buttocks while getting a great Pilates workout. With the support of the Pilates Bar, you can perform Pilates movements with the right alignment and form. With Pilates Bar Kicks, you can build your muscles while improving your coordination, flexibility, and balance.

Your legs and buttocks will be toned by the excellent Pilates exercise known as Pilates Bar Kicks. Since the Pilates Bar makes it simpler for you to perform Pilates exercises with proper form and alignment, Pilates Bar Kicks are a great method to improve your balance, coordination, and flexibility. For those looking to supplement their Pilates training routine, Pilates Bar Kicks are a great alternative because they help build muscle.

Regardless matter your level of experience; Pilates Bar Kicks is a terrific way to improve your training routine.

Pilates Bar and Steps

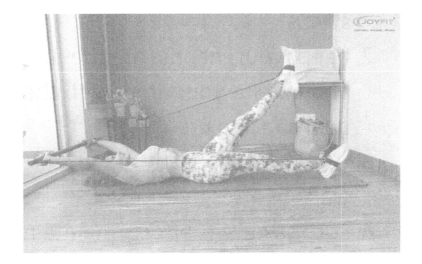

Steps are an excellent abs exercise for developing strength and tone. It is remarkably similar to ascending stairs. You simply lay on your back in this situation.

How to do:

1. Lay flat on your back and insert your feet into the foot straps.
2. Keep your hands on the bar and extend your arms with the palms facing up.
3. Lift each leg separately to start walking after that.
4. For maximum effect, maintain one leg in the highest position for 60 seconds.

Use three sets of 12 repetitions to achieve the best results.

Lifting the Leg with A Bar

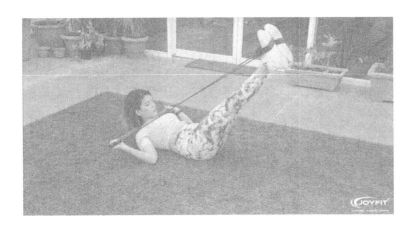

Your abs will tone up as a result of lifting the leg to workout the muscles surrounding your body's core.

How to do:

1. Place a Pilates bar beneath your arms and foot straps

under your feet while lying on your back.

2. Make sure to keep your legs straight and pointing up.

3. Keeping your arms straight, hold the Bar above your head. Make sure the tubing is put under sufficient pressure.

4. You should elevate one leg at a time higher than 45 degrees while keeping your toes tucked under the foot straps.

5. After maintaining this position for at least 60 seconds on each leg, switch sides.

Work 12 times on each side across three sets. Keep performing this workout and you'll see improvements in two weeks!

Bicep Curls

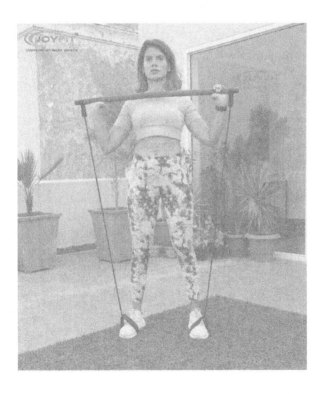

Bicep curls work particularly effectively on the lengthy head of your biceps.

How to do:

1. Hold on to the bar and insert your feet into the foot straps.
2. The bicep muscles contract more forcefully while the palms remain downward.
3. As you bend your elbows at a 90-degree angle, maintaining your upper arm steady, curl your hands towards your shoulder without moving your shoulders or hips.

4. Keep your legs straight when doing this exercise for the best benefits!

For best results, complete three sets of 12 repetitions on each side. You'll notice a difference in a week!

Air Cycling

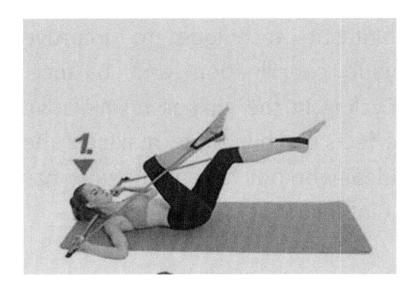

Would you wish to improve your Pilates posture? So, Pilates Bar The ideal workout for you might be air cycling. This unique exercise method combines the benefits of Pilates with the cardio workout of cycling while hanging in the air!

Bar workout a great full body exercise, air cycling works all of the major muscle groups. It's also a fantastic technique to improve your coordination and balance. Cycling in the air has no negative effects on your joints, making it the ideal workout for anyone who has joint injuries or issues.

If you're looking for a challenging and pleasant way to enhance your Pilates practice, Pilates Bar Cycling in the Air is definitely worth giving a shot.

Bar Squats

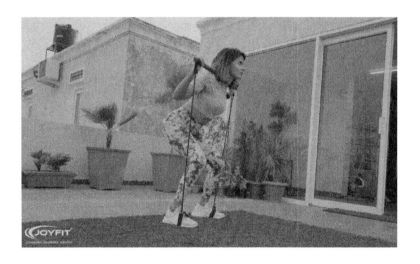

This exercise is a great way to begin your Pilates bar training program. It is a great place to start because it promotes the growth of muscles, especially the glutes.

How to do:

1. Your shoulders should be in front of the bar. Make sure that when you are standing, your feet are wider than hip-width apart.
2. Set the foot strap securely on your feet.
3. With your knees bent, squat down and stay there for at least 60 seconds.

Do this exercise three times for a total of 12 reps. Your results will get better after a few weeks.

Bar Lunges

Lunges are a great exercise for enlarging and toning the legs. The growth of the hamstrings, glutes, and core muscles is also greatly aided by them.

How to do:

1. Your shoulders should be in front of the bar.
2. Your feet should be hip-width apart.

3. Lunge forward while taking a step back to feel the stretch in your front thigh muscle.
4. In order to properly complete this exercise, your knee should be above your ankle.
5. Keep your body in this position for at least 60 seconds while holding on to the pole of the Pilates bar or, if necessary, any other nearby support point.
6. For this workout, do three sets of 12 reps on each side.

You'll begin to see outcomes within two weeks!

Overhead Press

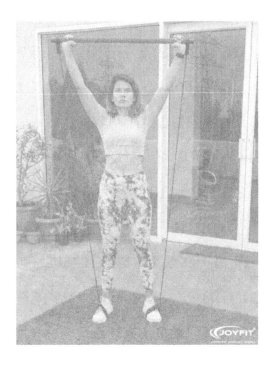

The shoulders and triceps benefit greatly from this exercise. A portion of your chest and your core muscles are also used. As a result, it meets the criteria for a compound exercise.

How to do:

1. As firmly as you are able, grasp the bar in front of you at shoulder height or higher.
2. Maintain straight elbows and upward-facing hands as you hoist the weight.
3. Bring your palms back down to the beginning position when the bands are too loose.

Perform three sets of 12 reps each, three times per day.

Plank in Reverse

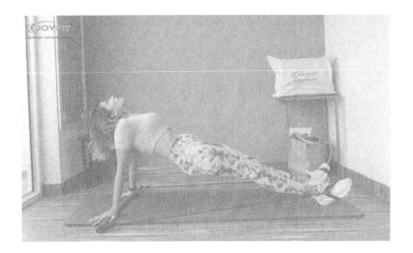

Your legs and core will benefit greatly from the reverse plank. Your lower back, thighs, hips, and abs will all be worked out.

How to Do

1. Your palms should be facing down while you hold the bar while lying on the ground.
2. Stretch your legs while securing your feet with the foot straps.
3. Utilize your hands, core, and feet to raise your body up.
4. Change legs after maintaining this position for at least 60 to 100 seconds.

You might get incredible outcomes with just 3 minutes of hold time per day.

Note: Pilates bar exercises are a terrific choice if you're searching for a workout that can enhance your posture, tone your muscles, and aid in calorie burning. Pilates bar exercises can enhance your coordination and mental wellness in addition to these advantages. Additionally recognized for lowering stress levels and boosting flexibility, Pilates bar movements. Pilates bar exercises are a great option if you want a workout that will provide you all of these advantages.

CONCLUSION

Several Positive Behaviors That Can Improve Your Lifestyle

Want to adopt a healthy lifestyle? Simply step outside of your comfort zone to adopt a healthy lifestyle. What exactly does it mean to leave your comfort zone? I don't wish to offend anyone, but in our society, a lot of people exhibit laziness when it comes to working. Whether we focus on a person's personal life, professional life, or everyday chores they complete, the job can be of any kind. They operate without enthusiasm and with no energy. They ultimately lead unhealthy lives as a result, which can cause a great deal of problems for them. One has claimed that in order to achieve something in life, one must step outside of their comfort zone.

If you want to succeed in life, you must put in the necessary time and effort. Don't be slow and lazy; time is money that, once spent, can never be retrieved. In order to avoid losing everything in life, try to accomplish everything in this brief amount of time. We'll talk about several positive habits that can improve your living. How can your living be made better? To lead a life that is ideal, adopt some positive behaviors. Check out some of the positive behaviors listed below to change your way of life.

Create a Positive Self-Image to Change Your Behavior

If you're serious about altering your way of life, you must develop a positive self-perception in order to change your habits. By making a few adjustments to your behaviors, this is the finest approach to improve your living. You must first assess yourself by being familiar with oneself. Knowing yourself is the first step to improving your life. Make life goals. Change everything that can be changed in order to develop into a nice person with aspirations. Don't forget to aim higher if you want to succeed in life. Make sure your success fits into your way of life. Setting a goal is all you need to do to enhance your lifestyle. If you make goals for yourself, your life will change for the better. The best method to improve your lifestyle is through this. You need to educate yourself on this. You can't have goals in life if you don't love who you are. To get better achievements, stop criticizing others and start expressing gratitude. Your strategy will change as a result, and you'll undoubtedly improve your way of life.

Focus on One Objective to Create Healthy Habits

Concentrating on a single objective at a time is another crucial aspect of creating excellent habits. Multitasking is encouraged, but focus on one activity at a time. Focusing on one item at a time will help you live a better life; it's a healthy habit that will help you succeed in life. Respectfully, you can improve your way of life by doing that. Don't divide your energy and try to accomplish one aim first; doing so will sap your energy. Instead, focus all of your efforts on one goal at a time. After you reach your goal, move on to the next. You'll form healthy behaviors this way.

Put Yourself First In Order To Improve Your Lifestyle

This appears to be an important point. Learn to value yourself in order to become a brave and self-assured person in life if you want to better your way of life. We notice that many people have the bad tendency of ignoring themselves, which is not a desirable habit to have. Never rush yourself, and always value your judgment. You will start to lose confidence as soon as you begin to underestimate yourself. To lose confidence is not a good thing! If you're serious about improving your way of life, start by loving yourself and avoiding hate. Be a responsible adult or share your opinions everywhere.

A Good Education Will Teach You Morals And Manners.

You need to be educated in order to have a healthy lifestyle. You become a good person through education, which teaches you ethics and manners. Both are beneficial for leading a better lifestyle. A good education will undoubtedly teach you morals and etiquette. While formal education should be prioritized first, self-education is the best form of education there is. By engaging in self-education, you can learn so much. Simply put, developing good morals and etiquette will make you a better person.

Belief in Yourself to Boost Confidence

A solid education always boosts your confidence. Without a doubt, education increases confidence, therefore never stop believing in yourself. You can always develop your public speaking skills if you believe in yourself. The most effective way to enhance your lifestyle is through social confidence. Therefore, starting to trust oneself is the only way to increase your confidence. Your lack of self-confidence will make you frail. You should never strive to lead a life of failure. Therefore, never give up and always act with confidence.

How to Deal with Difficult Situations

You must constantly develop effective situational management skills if you want to change your way of life. Furthermore, you must master this art if you want to better your way of life. Undoubtedly, managing a difficult situation is a skill that hardly everyone possesses. Tragedies are a part of life and can put anyone in danger, thus handling the issue requires a cool head. One needs to be equipped for difficult times. One should learn how to manage difficult circumstances in addition to preparing for them. Keep your emotions and wrath under control. Keep your cool to control the situation effectively. This will inevitably boost your self-confidence. You should create this habit in order to improve your living.

You have a plethora of options for enhancing your way of life. Never underestimate yourself in life because everyone wants to live a healthy lifestyle. Every day, compete with yourself in the mirror. You struggle alone in life; you are the only one standing between you and your objectives. Take care! Furthermore, always prioritize healthy eating in life to improve your lifestyle. Keep in mind that eating well will keep you motivated to achieve your goals.

Printed in Great Britain
by Amazon

40380979R00036